Resistance Band Exercise Easy Guide for Beginners

Incorporating Resistance Band Exercise into Daily Routines

By

Fyvie Greig

Copyright@2023

Table of Contents

CHAPTER 1

Introduction

1.1 What are Resistance Bands?

Resistance bands are versatile fitness tools made of elastic materials designed to provide resistance during exercise. They offer a portable, affordable, and effective way to engage in strength training, rehabilitation, and flexibility exercises. These bands come in various lengths, thicknesses, and resistance levels, catering to individuals of different fitness levels, from beginners to advanced athletes.

Key Characteristics:

- **Elasticity:** Resistance bands are made from durable rubber or latex and can stretch to varying degrees based on their thickness and composition.

- **Adjustable Resistance:** Their resistance level can be adjusted by altering the band's length, grip, or combining multiple bands to increase resistance.

- **Portability:** They are lightweight and easy to carry, making them suitable for home workouts, travel, or gym sessions.

- **Versatility:** These bands offer a wide range of exercises targeting different muscle groups, allowing for a full-body workout.

- **Low Impact:** They provide a low-impact alternative to free weights, reducing the risk of joint strain or injury while still building strength and endurance.

Uses of Resistance Bands:

1. **Strength Training:** They help build and tone muscles, mimicking the resistance provided by traditional weights.

2. **Rehabilitation:** Often used in physical therapy for injury rehabilitation due to their gentle resistance and ability to isolate specific muscle groups.

3. **Flexibility and Mobility:** Resistance bands assist in stretching exercises, improving flexibility and enhancing joint mobility.

4. **Functional Training:** They support functional movements, replicating real-life motions and engaging multiple muscle groups simultaneously.

5. **Supplementary Training:** They can complement other forms of exercise, such as yoga, Pilates, or CrossFit, by adding resistance to bodyweight exercises.

1.2 Types of Resistance Bands

a. Tube Bands:

- **Design:** These bands resemble hollow tubes with handles on either end, providing a firm grip during exercises.

- **Variability:** They come in various resistance levels, often color-coded for easy identification.

- **Versatility:** Tube bands offer a wide range of exercises for both upper and lower body workouts.

b. Loop Bands:

- **Structure:** Loop bands form closed loops without handles, providing resistance by wrapping around or placing them on body parts.

- **Usage:** They are popular for lower body exercises like squats, lunges, and glute activation.

- **Variable Resistance:** Loop bands vary in thickness, offering different resistance levels based on their size and material.

c. Therapy Bands:

- **Characteristics:** These bands are flat, wide, and typically made of latex or rubber, catering to rehabilitation and gentle strength training.

- **Flexibility:** Therapy bands offer gradual resistance, making them suitable for those recovering from injuries or needing light resistance.

d. Figure-8 Bands:

- **Structure:** These bands are shaped like a figure-eight, providing a more secure grip during exercises.

- **Focus:** They are often used for upper body workouts, particularly targeting the arms, chest, and shoulders.

e. Superbands:

- **Features:** Superbands are longer and thicker bands designed to offer heavier resistance compared to other types.

- **Applications:** They are commonly used for powerlifting, assisted pull-ups, and adding substantial resistance to exercises.

Understanding the different types of resistance bands allows individuals to select the appropriate band based on their fitness goals, desired resistance level, and targeted muscle groups. Experimenting with various bands can also add diversity and challenge to workout routines, ensuring continuous progress and adaptation.

Resistance bands, with their adaptability and effectiveness, have become integral tools in fitness programs worldwide, catering to diverse populations seeking strength, flexibility, and overall wellness.

Would you like more information on any specific aspect of resistance bands?

1.3 Benefits of Using Resistance Bands

Resistance bands offer a multitude of advantages, making them a popular choice for fitness enthusiasts, athletes, and those engaged in rehabilitation programs. Here are the key benefits:

1. Versatility:

- **Multiple Exercises:** Bands facilitate a wide range of exercises targeting various muscle groups, allowing for a comprehensive full-body workout.

- **Adaptable Resistance:** Bands come in different resistance levels, offering scalability for beginners to advanced users.

2. Portability and Convenience:

- **Compact:** They are lightweight and portable, making them suitable for home workouts, travel, or exercising outdoors.

- **Space Efficient:** Unlike bulky gym equipment, resistance bands require minimal storage space.

3. Joint-Friendly and Low-Impact:

- **Reduced Strain:** Bands provide constant tension without the jarring impact associated with heavy weights, reducing the risk of joint strain or injury.

- **Suitable for Rehabilitation:** Their gentle resistance makes them ideal for individuals recovering from injuries or undergoing rehabilitation.

4. Enhances Strength and Muscle Tone:

- **Muscle Engagement:** Bands create resistance throughout the entire movement, engaging muscles both concentrically and eccentrically, leading to improved strength and muscle tone.

- **Targeted Workouts:** They allow for isolated muscle targeting, helping in strengthening weaker muscle groups.

5. Improves Flexibility and Mobility:

- **Stretching Aid:** Bands assist in stretching exercises, enhancing flexibility, and promoting better range of motion in joints.

- **Joint Health:** Regular use can help alleviate stiffness and improve overall joint mobility.

6. Suitable for All Fitness Levels:

- **Scalable Resistance:** Bands are adaptable, allowing users to start with lighter resistance and progressively increase intensity as strength improves.

- **Beginner-Friendly:** They are accessible to beginners due to their ease of use and lower risk of injury.

7. Cost-Effective Fitness Solution:

- **Affordability:** Compared to traditional gym equipment, resistance bands are relatively inexpensive while offering a variety of exercises and benefits.

8. Additional Functional Training:

- **Functional Movements:** Bands facilitate functional training, replicating natural movements, and assisting in improving overall functional fitness.

1.4 Safety Precautions and Considerations

While resistance bands are generally safe and user-friendly, it's essential to observe certain safety precautions:

1. Band Inspection:

- **Regular Check:** Inspect bands for any tears, wear, or damage before each use. Replace damaged bands to avoid injury.

2. Proper Form and Technique:

- **Correct Posture:** Maintain proper form during exercises to prevent strains or injuries. Focus on controlled movements.

- **Proper Anchoring:** Securely anchor the bands to a stable surface or object to avoid snapping or unexpected movements.

3. Gradual Progression:

- **Start Light:** Beginners should start with lighter resistance and gradually progress to higher levels to avoid overexertion or muscle strain.

4. Avoid Overstretching:

- **Controlled Stretch:** Avoid overstretching bands beyond their limit to prevent them from snapping back and causing injury.

5. Supervision for Beginners:

- **Guidance:** Beginners or those new to resistance bands should seek guidance from fitness professionals to learn proper techniques and exercises.

6. Health Considerations:

- **Consultation:** Individuals with pre-existing medical conditions or injuries should consult a healthcare professional before starting a resistance band workout routine.

CHAPTER 2

Getting Started with Resistance Bands

2.1 Selecting the Right Resistance Band

Choosing the appropriate resistance band is crucial for an effective and safe workout. Here's how to select the right band:

1. Determine Fitness Level:

- **Beginners:** Start with lighter resistance bands to get accustomed to the movements and gradually increase resistance.

- **Intermediate/Advanced:** Those with experience can opt for bands with higher resistance levels for more challenging workouts.

2. Consider Band Types:

- **Tube Bands:** Offer various resistance levels with handles, suitable for both upper and lower body workouts.

- **Loop Bands:** Ideal for lower body exercises like squats and glute activation, available in different thicknesses indicating resistance.

- **Therapy Bands:** Provide lighter resistance, perfect for rehabilitation or those requiring gentle strength training.

- **Figure-8 Bands and Superbands:** These provide specific forms of resistance and are typically used for targeted exercises.

3. Resistance Level:

- **Color Coding:** Many bands are color-coded to signify resistance levels. For instance, yellow might indicate light resistance, while black might represent heavy resistance.

- **Test Resistance:** Some brands specify resistance in pounds or kilograms. Testing the resistance by stretching the band can help determine its suitability.

4. Length and Material:

- **Length Variation:** Bands come in different lengths; longer bands can offer more versatility in exercises.

- **Material Quality:** Look for durable bands made from high-quality latex or rubber to ensure longevity and safety during workouts.

5. Personal Goals and Exercises:

- **Exercise Specificity:** Consider the exercises you plan to perform. Different bands suit various exercises, so choose accordingly.

- **Full-Body or Targeted Workouts:** Decide if you want a band for full-body workouts or for targeting specific muscle groups.

6. Set or Individual Bands:

- **Sets:** Some bands are sold in sets with varying resistance levels, providing options for different exercises and progressions.

- **Individual Bands:** Purchasing bands individually allows customization based on specific resistance needs.

2.2 Understanding Resistance Band Terminology

1. Resistance Level:

- **Light, Medium, Heavy:** Bands are often categorized by these levels, indicating the amount of resistance they provide.

2. Loop Band Sizes:

- **Light to Heavy:** Loop bands come in different sizes/thicknesses, usually identified by colors or resistance levels (e.g., light, medium, heavy).

3. Handles, Anchors, and Accessories:

- **Handles:** Found on tube bands, they provide grip during exercises and come in various designs for comfort and usability.

- **Anchors:** Some bands have anchor points or attachments for securing to door frames, poles, or other stable structures.

- **Accessories:** Some sets may include additional items like ankle straps, door anchors, or instructional materials.

4. Material Quality and Composition:

- **Latex or Rubber:** Most bands are made from these materials. Higher-quality latex or rubber bands tend to be more durable and resistant to snapping.

5. Length and Width:

- **Length:** Longer bands offer more versatility in exercises, especially for standing or full-body movements.

- **Width:** Wider bands may provide more resistance due to increased surface area.

6. Elasticity and Stretch:

- **Elasticity:** Bands vary in stretchability. Understanding the elasticity helps determine how much resistance will be experienced during exercises.

7. Band Care and Maintenance:

- **Cleaning:** Instructions for cleaning and maintaining bands vary. Some may need to be wiped with a damp cloth, while others are washable.

Understanding these terminologies assists in making informed decisions when purchasing resistance bands and ensures you select the right bands for your fitness level, goals, and intended workout routines. Always follow manufacturer guidelines for safe usage and maintenance of your resistance bands.

2.3 Proper Set-Up and Handling of Resistance Bands

1. Anchoring:

- **Secure Attachment:** For tube bands with anchors, ensure they are firmly attached to a stable structure like a door frame, pole, or an anchor specifically designed for bands.

- **Stability Check:** Verify the anchor's stability to prevent accidents or bands snapping back unexpectedly during exercises.

2. Band Handling:

- **Grip and Positioning:** Hold the bands securely, ensuring proper grip and positioning to maintain control throughout the movement.

- **Avoid Sharp Edges:** Prevent bands from coming into contact with sharp or abrasive surfaces that could cause damage or weaken the material.

3. Band Inspection:

- **Regular Checks:** Before each use, inspect bands for any tears, wear, or signs of damage. Replace damaged bands promptly to prevent accidents.

4. Proper Form:

- **Alignment:** Maintain proper body alignment and posture during exercises to prevent strain or injury.

- **Controlled Movements:** Perform exercises with controlled and deliberate movements to maximize effectiveness and safety.

5. Understanding Resistance:

- **Gradual Increase:** Start with a comfortable resistance level and gradually increase it as strength improves.

- **Maintaining Tension:** Maintain tension in the band throughout the exercise to ensure consistent resistance.

6. Supervision for Beginners:

- **Guidance:** Beginners should seek guidance from fitness professionals to learn proper handling techniques and exercise execution.

2.4 Warm-Up and Stretching Exercises

1. Dynamic Warm-Up:

- **Cardiovascular Warm-Up:** Engage in light cardiovascular activity such as jogging or jumping jacks for 5-10 minutes to increase heart rate and blood flow.

- **Joint Mobility:** Perform dynamic stretches that involve controlled movements to warm up major muscle groups and joints.

2. Specific Warm-Up with Resistance Bands:

- **Light Resistance:** Use a lighter resistance band to perform dynamic movements that mimic the exercises planned for the workout.

- **Range of Motion:** Focus on moving through the full range of motion for each exercise to prepare the muscles and joints.

3. Stretching Exercises:

- **Targeted Stretching:** Utilize resistance bands for stretching exercises after the warm-up or workout to enhance flexibility.

- **Hold and Breathe:** Hold each stretch for 15-30 seconds while maintaining steady breathing. Avoid bouncing.

4. Major Muscle Groups:

- **Full-Body Approach:** Include stretches targeting major muscle groups like quadriceps, hamstrings, calves, chest, back, shoulders, and hips.

- **Post-Workout Stretching:** Perform static stretches using bands to aid in muscle recovery and reduce post-exercise soreness.

5. Cooling Down:

- **Gradual Decrease in Intensity:** After the workout, gradually reduce the intensity of exercises before concluding the session.

- **Foam Rolling:** Consider using a foam roller or self-massage techniques for myofascial release to further aid in recovery.

6. Hydration and Rest:

- **Stay Hydrated:** Drink water before, during, and after the workout to maintain hydration levels.

- **Rest and Recovery:** Allow the body proper time to recover between workouts to prevent overuse injuries.

By adhering to proper set-up techniques and handling practices, individuals can ensure safe and effective use of resistance bands during exercises. Incorporating warm-up, stretching, and cooldown routines helps prepare the body, prevent injury, and optimize the benefits of resistance band workouts. Always listen to

your body and avoid pushing beyond your
limits to maintain a safe and enjoyable
fitness experience.

CHAPTER 3

Upper Body Exercises

3.1 Bicep Curls

Setup:

1. Stand with both feet on the resistance band, ensuring it's evenly distributed under both feet.

2. Grasp the handles or ends of the band, palms facing upward, keeping elbows close to your sides.

Execution:

1. With controlled movements, curl your hands toward your shoulders while keeping your upper arms stationary.

2. Squeeze your biceps at the top of the movement, then slowly lower back to the starting position.

3. Maintain tension on the band throughout the exercise.

Variations:

- *Single-Arm Curls:* Perform curls with one arm at a time, focusing on each bicep individually.

- *Hammer Curls:* Palms face each other throughout the movement, engaging both the biceps and forearms.

3.2 Shoulder Press

Setup:

1. Stand on the resistance band with feet shoulder-width apart.

2. Hold the handles or band ends at shoulder height, elbows bent, palms facing forward.

Execution:

1. Press the bands upward, straightening your arms overhead without locking your elbows.

2. Slowly return to the starting position, controlling the band's resistance.

Variations:

- *Arnold Press:* Start with palms facing you, rotate them outward as you press, then bring them back to the starting position while rotating back inward.

- *Seated Shoulder Press:* Sit on a chair or bench and perform the same movement, focusing on stabilizing your core.

3.3 Tricep Extensions

Setup:

1. Stand with one foot in the middle of the band, holding the band's

other end behind your back with the same-side hand.

2. Position your free hand over your shoulder and grasp the band, ensuring it's taut.

Execution:

1. Extend your arm overhead, straightening it while keeping your upper arm close to your head.

2. Slowly return to the starting position, maintaining tension on the band throughout the movement.

Variations:

- *Single-Arm Extensions:* Perform the exercise with one arm at a time, focusing on each tricep individually.

- *Overhead Tricep Extensions:* Use both hands to hold the band overhead and extend both arms upward, targeting both triceps simultaneously.

These upper body exercises utilizing resistance bands effectively target various muscle groups, offering a challenging workout while allowing for control over resistance levels. Ensure proper form and controlled movements for optimal results and to avoid any risk of injury.

3.4 Chest Press

Setup:

1. Secure the resistance band around a stable anchor behind you at chest height.

2. Hold the handles or ends of the band, facing away from the anchor, with arms extended in front at chest level.

Execution:

1. Push the bands forward, extending your arms in front of you.

2. Slowly return to the starting position, maintaining control over the band's resistance and keeping your elbows slightly bent.

Variations:

- *Single-Arm Chest Press:* Perform the press with one arm at a time to focus on each side of the chest independently.

- *Incline Chest Press:* Adjust the anchor point to a higher position to simulate an incline press, targeting the upper chest.

3.5 Back Rows

Setup:

1. Secure the band to a fixed point in front of you at waist height.

2. Hold the handles or ends, step back to create tension, and bend your

knees slightly while keeping your back straight.

Execution:

1. Pull the bands towards your waist by retracting your shoulder blades and bending your elbows.

2. Slowly return to the starting position, maintaining tension on the band throughout the movement.

Variations:

- *Wide Grip Rows:* Adjust hand positioning wider than shoulder-width to engage different back muscles.

- *Single-Arm Rows:* Perform the exercise one arm at a time for unilateral engagement and balance.

3.6 Exercises for the Deltoids

a. Lateral Raises

Setup:

1. Stand on the band with feet shoulder-width apart, holding the handles or band ends by your sides, palms facing inward.

Execution:

1. Raise your arms to the sides until they're parallel to the floor, keeping a slight bend in the elbows.

2. Slowly lower your arms back to the starting position, controlling the band's resistance.

Variations:

*   *Front Raises:* Perform a similar movement but raise your arms in front of you, targeting the front deltoids.

b. Rear Delt Flyes

Setup:

1. Stand on the band, bend forward slightly, holding the handles or band ends in front of your legs, palms facing each other.

Execution:

1. Lift your arms out to the sides, keeping elbows slightly bent, until they're parallel to the floor.

2. Slowly lower your arms back to the starting position while maintaining tension on the band.

Variations:

- *Seated Rear Delt Flyes:* Perform the exercise while seated on a chair or bench to isolate the rear deltoids.

These exercises effectively engage the chest, back, and deltoid muscles using resistance bands. Focus on proper form, controlled movements, and adjusting the band's resistance to suit your fitness level for a challenging and effective upper body workout.

CHAPTER 4

Lower Body Exercises

4.1 Squats

Setup:

1. Place the band under both feet, positioning your feet shoulder-width apart.

2. Hold the handles or band ends at shoulder height, crossing the bands in front of you and grasping them.

Execution:

1. Lower into a squat by bending your knees and pushing your hips back, keeping your chest up and back straight.

2. Push through your heels to return to the starting position, keeping tension on the band throughout.

Variations:

- *Sumo Squats:* Widen your stance and turn your toes out, targeting inner thighs.

- *Pulse Squats:* Hold the squat position and perform small pulsing movements to intensify the workout.

4.2 Lunges

Setup:

1. Stand on the band with one foot, bringing the other foot back to create tension.

2. Hold the handles or band ends at your sides or place them on your shoulders.

Execution:

1. Lower your body by bending both
    knees until your back knee is just
    above the ground.

2. Push through the front heel to
    return to the starting position,
    maintaining tension on the band.

Variations:

- *Reverse Lunges:* Step backward
  into the lunge instead of forward,
  engaging different muscles.

- *Walking Lunges:* Perform lunges
  while walking forward, alternating
  legs with each step.

4.3 Leg Press

Setup:

1. Sit on the floor or a bench and loop
    the band around the bottom of one
    foot.

2. Hold the band securely with both hands, positioning your foot against the band.

Execution:

1. Push your foot forward against the band, extending your leg fully while keeping your back straight.

2. Return to the starting position, maintaining tension on the band throughout the movement.

Variations:

- *Single-Leg Press:* Perform the exercise one leg at a time for unilateral engagement and balance.

- *Seated Leg Press:* Sit on a chair or bench and press against the band, focusing on stability and control.

These lower body exercises effectively target the quadriceps, hamstrings, glutes, and calf muscles using resistance bands. Remember to maintain proper form, control the movement, and adjust the band's resistance to suit your fitness level for a challenging and productive lower body workout.

4.4 Glute Bridges

Setup:

1. Lie on your back with knees bent and feet flat on the floor.

2. Place the resistance band just above your knees and secure it in place.

Execution:

1. Lift your hips off the ground, squeezing your glutes at the top of the movement.

2. Lower your hips back down without resting them on the floor and repeat.

Variations:

*   *Single-Leg Glute Bridges:* Extend one leg straight up while

performing the bridge with the other leg, focusing on one side at a time.

- *Elevated Glute Bridges:* Place your feet on an elevated surface (e.g., bench) to increase the range of motion.

4.5 Calf Raises

Setup:

1. Stand on the resistance band with feet shoulder-width apart.

2. Hold the handles or band ends at your sides or place them on your shoulders.

Execution:

1. Rise up onto the balls of your feet, lifting your heels as high as possible.

2. Lower your heels back down,
    keeping tension on the band
    throughout the movement.

Variations:

- *Single-Leg Calf Raises:* Perform
  the exercise on one leg at a time,
  focusing on each calf individually.

- *Seated Calf Raises:* Sit on a chair
  with the band under the balls of
  your feet and perform the raises
  from a seated position.

4.6 Outer Thigh Abduction

Setup:

1. Lie on your side with legs extended
    and the band placed around your
    thighs just above the knees.

2. Prop yourself up on your elbow or
    hand for support.

Execution:

1. Lift the top leg upward against the resistance band, keeping the foot flexed.

2. Lower the leg back down slowly without completely relaxing the tension on the band.

Variations:

- *Side-Lying Clamshell:* Bend your knees slightly and open your top knee while keeping your feet together, targeting the outer thighs and glutes.

These exercises specifically target the glutes, hamstrings, calves, and outer thigh muscles using resistance bands. Focus on form, engage the targeted muscles, and control the band's resistance for an effective lower body workout. Adjust the band's tension as needed to match your fitness level and ensure proper muscle engagement.

CHAPTER 5

Core Exercises

5.1 Russian Twists

Definition and Technique

Russian Twists are a dynamic core exercise that targets the obliques and the entire abdominal region. To perform this exercise:

1. Start by sitting on the floor with your knees bent and feet flat.

2. Lean back slightly, maintaining a straight spine.

3. Hold a weight or medicine ball with both hands, and lift your feet off the ground.

4. Twist your torso to one side, bringing the weight beside you.

5. Return to the center and twist to the other side.

Muscles Targeted

- **Obliques:** Russian Twists primarily engage the internal and external obliques, promoting waistline definition.

- **Rectus Abdominis:** The twisting motion activates the rectus abdominis, contributing to overall core strength.

- **Transverse Abdominis:** Stabilizes the spine and enhances core stability.

Variations and Progressions

- *Weighted Russian Twists:* Increase resistance by holding a heavier weight.

- *Russian Twist with Leg Raise:* Lift one leg off the ground during the twist for added difficulty.

5.2 Woodchoppers

Definition and Technique

Woodchoppers mimic the motion of chopping wood and are highly effective for targeting the obliques and core muscles:

1. Stand with feet shoulder-width apart, holding a resistance band or cable with both hands.

2. Rotate your torso diagonally, bringing the band or cable across your body.

3. Engage your core and control the movement as you return to the starting position.

Muscles Targeted

- **Obliques:** Woodchoppers emphasize oblique muscles, enhancing side-to-side functional strength.

- **Rectus Abdominis:** The twisting and chopping motion engages the entire abdominal region.

- **Back Muscles:** Woodchoppers engage the lower and upper back, promoting a well-rounded core workout.

Variations and Progressions

- *High to Low Woodchopper:* Start the movement with the hands high and bring them down diagonally.

- *Medicine Ball Woodchopper:* Use a medicine ball for added resistance.

5.3 Plank Variations

Definition and Technique

Planks are a fundamental core exercise, and variations add complexity to challenge different muscle groups:

1. **Traditional Plank:**

- Start in a push-up position with elbows directly beneath your shoulders.

- Maintain a straight line from head to heels, engaging your core.

2. **Side Plank:**

- Rotate to one side, balancing on one elbow and the side of your foot.

- Keep your body in a straight line, engaging the obliques.

3. **Plank with Leg Lift:**

- From the traditional plank, lift one leg off the ground, engaging the glutes and lower abdominals.

Muscles Targeted

- **Rectus Abdominis:** Planks engage the entire abdominal region, promoting overall core stability.

- **Obliques:** Side planks specifically target the side muscles, enhancing waistline definition.

- **Transverse Abdominis:** Activated to stabilize the spine and maintain proper form.

Variations and Progressions

- *Dynamic Plank:* Incorporate small hip dips or knee taps to make the plank dynamic.

- *Plank with Alternating Arm and Leg Lifts:* Lift opposite arm and leg while maintaining the plank position.

Benefits of Incorporating These Core Exercises

1. **Improved Stability and Posture:** Russian Twists and Woodchoppers enhance rotational stability, contributing to better overall posture.

2. **Functional Strength:**
    Woodchoppers mimic real-world
    movements, promoting functional
    strength for daily activities.

3. **Versatility:** Plank variations
    provide a versatile core workout
    adaptable to various fitness levels
    and goals.

4. **Balanced Development:** Together,
    these exercises ensure a balanced
    development of the entire core,
    reducing the risk of muscle
    imbalances and injuries.

Incorporating these core exercises into
your fitness routine can lead to a stronger,
more stable core, with benefits extending
beyond aesthetic improvements to overall
functional fitness and injury prevention.
Remember to maintain proper form,
gradually progress in intensity, and consult
with a fitness professional if needed.

5.4 Bicycle Crunches

Bicycle crunches are a dynamic and effective abdominal exercise that engages multiple muscle groups. The technique involves:

1. Lie on your back, placing your hands behind your head and lifting your legs off the ground.

2. Bring your right elbow toward your left knee while simultaneously straightening your right leg.

3. Repeat the motion on the other side, creating a pedaling motion resembling riding a bicycle.

Muscles Targeted

- **Rectus Abdominis:** Bicycle crunches activate the entire abdominal region, particularly the rectus abdominis.

- **Obliques:** The twisting motion engages the internal and external obliques.

- **Hip Flexors:** Lifting the legs engages the hip flexor muscles.

Variations and Progressions

- *Slow Bicycle Crunches:* Perform the exercise with a slower, controlled tempo to increase time under tension.

- *Weighted Bicycle Crunches:* Hold a lightweight medicine ball or add ankle weights for added resistance.

5.5 Pallof Press

Definition and Technique

The Pallof Press is a functional core exercise that focuses on anti-rotation, enhancing stability and strength:

1. Attach a resistance band to a stationary object at chest height.

2. Stand perpendicular to the anchor point, holding the band with both hands at chest level.

3. Extend your arms fully, resisting the band's attempt to rotate your torso.

4. Hold for a few seconds before returning to the starting position.

Muscles Targeted

- **Transverse Abdominis:** Pallof Press engages the deep core muscles responsible for stabilizing the spine.

- **Obliques:** The anti-rotation aspect targets the internal and external obliques.

- **Rectus Abdominis:** Maintaining an upright position activates the rectus abdominis.

Variations and Progressions

- *Half-Kneeling Pallof Press:* Perform the exercise in a half-kneeling position to increase instability and challenge balance.

- *Single-Arm Pallof Press:* Focus on one side at a time, intensifying the anti-rotation demand.

Benefits of Incorporating These Core Exercises

1. **Complete Core Activation:** Bicycle crunches engage both the upper and lower abdominals, providing a comprehensive core workout.

2. **Enhanced Stability:** Pallof Press improves core stability, which is crucial for maintaining proper posture and preventing injuries.

3. **Versatility:** Both exercises offer variations that cater to different fitness levels and goals.

4. **Functional Strength:** The dynamic nature of bicycle crunches and the anti-rotational focus of Pallof Press contribute to functional strength transferable to daily activities.

Incorporating these core exercises into your fitness routine adds variety and targets different aspects of core strength. Remember to maintain proper form, control the movements, and gradually progress in intensity to maximize the benefits while minimizing the risk of injury. As always, consult with a fitness professional if you have any concerns or specific health conditions.

CHAPTER 6

Full Body and Functional Exercises

6.1 Resistance Band Deadlifts

Definition and Technique

Resistance Band Deadlifts are a compound exercise that targets the muscles in the lower back, glutes, hamstrings, and core:

1. Place the resistance band under your feet, positioning them shoulder-width apart.

2. Hold the band with both hands, keeping your palms facing your body.

3. Hinge at your hips, keeping your back straight, and bend your knees slightly.

4. Engage your core and lift your torso to a fully upright position, extending your hips and knees.

Muscles Targeted

- **Erector Spinae:** The muscles along the spine are engaged in maintaining an upright posture.

- **Gluteus Maximus:** Resistance Band Deadlifts activate the glutes, promoting hip extension.

- **Hamstrings:** The bending at the knees engages the hamstrings.

- **Core Muscles:** Keeping the core engaged stabilizes the spine throughout the movement.

Variations and Progressions

- *Single-Leg Resistance Band Deadlifts:* Lift one leg off the ground during the deadlift for increased stability and balance challenge.

- *Sumo Stance Deadlifts:* Widen your stance for a sumo deadlift variation, targeting the inner thighs more intensely.

6.2 Standing Rows

Definition and Technique

Standing Rows with resistance bands target the muscles in the upper back, shoulders, and arms:

1. Secure the resistance band at chest height, or use a door anchor for versatility.

2. Stand facing the anchor point, holding the band with both hands.

3. Pull the band toward your chest, squeezing your shoulder blades together.

4. Keep your elbows close to your body and maintain a controlled motion.

Muscles Targeted

- **Latissimus Dorsi:** Standing Rows effectively target the large muscles of the upper back.

- **Rhomboids:** Squeezing the shoulder blades together activates the rhomboid muscles.

- **Deltoids:** The shoulders are engaged throughout the pulling motion.

- **Biceps:** The biceps are involved as secondary muscles in the rowing movement.

Variations and Progressions

- *Underhand Grip Rows:* Change your grip to underhand to emphasize the biceps and lower traps.

- *Single-Arm Standing Rows:* Perform the exercise with one arm at a time to address muscle imbalances.

Benefits of Full Body and Functional Exercises

1. **Efficient Workouts:** Both Resistance Band Deadlifts and Standing Rows engage multiple muscle groups, making them time-efficient for full-body workouts.

2. **Functional Movement Patterns:** These exercises mimic real-world movements, promoting functional strength and coordination.

3. **Scalability:** The resistance band's versatility allows for easy adjustment of resistance levels, accommodating various fitness levels.

4. **Core Engagement:** Both exercises require core stabilization, contributing to overall core strength.

Incorporating full-body and functional exercises like Resistance Band Deadlifts and Standing Rows into your routine not only enhances muscle development but also supports functional fitness, making daily activities easier and more efficient. Always prioritize proper form, start with an appropriate resistance level, and progress gradually to maximize the benefits while minimizing the risk of injury. If you have any concerns or pre-existing conditions, consult with a fitness professional before adding new exercises to your routine.

6.3 Push-Pull Exercises

Push-pull exercises are a category of compound movements that involve both pushing and pulling motions. This balanced approach helps target various muscle groups, promoting overall strength and muscle development.

Examples of Push-Pull Exercises

6.3.1 Push-Up Variations

- *Traditional Push-Up:* Targets the chest, shoulders, triceps, and core.

- *Wide Grip Push-Up:* Emphasizes the chest and outer part of the pectoral muscles.

- *Diamond Push-Up:* Focuses on the triceps and inner chest.

6.3.2 Bent-Over Rows

- *Barbell Bent-Over Rows:* Targets the upper back, lats, and biceps.

- *Dumbbell Bent-Over Rows:* Provides unilateral engagement, addressing muscle imbalances.

6.3.3 Overhead Press

- *Barbell Overhead Press:* Engages the shoulders, triceps, and upper back.

- *Dumbbell Overhead Press:* Enhances stability by isolating each arm.

Benefits of Push-Pull Exercises

1. **Muscle Balance:** Push-pull exercises help maintain a balanced development of opposing muscle groups, reducing the risk of imbalances and injuries.

2. **Efficient Workouts:** Combining pushing and pulling movements in a workout optimizes time and energy expenditure.

3. **Joint Health:** The balanced approach promotes joint health by evenly distributing stress across various joints.

6.4 Total Body Circuit Training

Total body circuit training involves performing a series of exercises in a circuit format, targeting different muscle groups and incorporating both strength and cardiovascular components.

Components of a Total Body Circuit

6.4.1 Strength Exercises

- *Resistance Band Squats:* Targets the lower body, including quads, hamstrings, and glutes.

- *Push-Ups:* Engages the chest, shoulders, triceps, and core.

- *Standing Rows with Resistance Bands:* Targets the upper back and biceps.

6.4.2 Cardiovascular Exercises

- *Jumping Jacks:* Elevates heart rate and improves cardiovascular endurance.

- *High Knees:* Engages the lower body while providing a cardiovascular boost.

- *Mountain Climbers:* Targets the core and elevates heart rate.

6.4.3 Flexibility and Mobility

- *Dynamic Lunges:* Enhances flexibility and engages the lower body.

- *Arm Circles:* Improves shoulder mobility and flexibility.

Benefits of Total Body Circuit Training

1. **Efficient Full-Body Workout:** Targets multiple muscle groups in one session.

2. **Calorie Burn:** Combines strength and cardiovascular exercises for effective calorie expenditure.

3. **Time Savings:** Ideal for individuals with limited time, providing a comprehensive workout in a shorter duration.

4. **Adaptability:** Can be modified for various fitness levels by adjusting exercise intensity and rest periods.

Incorporating push-pull exercises and total body circuit training into your fitness routine provides a well-rounded approach, addressing strength, cardiovascular fitness, and overall functional movement. Customize the intensity and exercises based on your fitness level and goals, and always prioritize proper form and safety during workouts. If you have any health concerns, consider consulting with a fitness professional before starting a new exercise program.

CHAPTER 7

Advanced Techniques and Variations

7.1 Adding Resistance Bands to Traditional Exercises

Adding resistance bands to traditional exercises is a method of increasing the intensity and challenge of familiar movements by incorporating the variable resistance provided by the bands. This technique is widely used to enhance muscle engagement, promote muscle endurance, and break through plateaus in strength training.

Examples of Exercises with Resistance Bands

7.1.1 Squats with Resistance Bands

- *Setup:* Place the resistance band around your thighs, just above the knees.

- *Execution:* Perform squats as usual, feeling the resistance from the band, particularly in the outer thighs.

7.1.2 Bench Press with Resistance Bands

- *Setup:* Attach resistance bands to the sides of the barbell and anchor them beneath the bench.

- *Execution:* As you lift the barbell during a bench press, the resistance bands add tension, making the movement more challenging at the top.

7.1.3 Deadlifts with Resistance Bands

- *Setup:* Loop the resistance band around the barbell and anchor it to the ground.

- *Execution:* As you lift the barbell, the band adds resistance, increasing the difficulty at the top of the deadlift.

Benefits of Adding Resistance Bands

1. **Variable Resistance:** Resistance bands provide more resistance as they are stretched, creating a variable load that challenges muscles throughout the entire range of motion.

2. **Increased Muscle Activation:** Adding bands activates stabilizing muscles and engages different muscle fibers, leading to enhanced muscle activation and development.

3. **Joint-Friendly Resistance:** The accommodating resistance of bands reduces stress on joints during certain phases of exercises, promoting joint health.

7.2 Resistance Band Progressions

Resistance band progressions involve gradually increasing the difficulty of exercises by using bands with higher resistance levels, challenging the muscles to adapt and grow stronger over time. This technique is essential for individuals looking to continually progress in their fitness journey.

Progression Examples

7.2.1 Bicep Curls with Increasing Resistance

- *Beginner:* Start with a light resistance band and perform standard bicep curls.

- *Intermediate:* Progress to a medium resistance band, increasing the challenge.

- *Advanced:* Use a heavy resistance band or combine multiple bands for a more intense workout.

7.2.2 Pull-Ups with Assisted Resistance Bands

- *Beginner:* Use a thick resistance band for assistance, looping it around the pull-up bar and placing a foot or knee in it.

- *Intermediate:* Gradually switch to thinner bands or reduce the assistance provided by the band.

- *Advanced:* Perform unassisted pull-ups as strength improves.

7.2.3 Lateral Band Walks with Increasing Tension

- *Beginner:* Start with a light resistance band around your thighs.

- *Intermediate:* Progress to a band with higher tension.

- *Advanced:* Use a heavier band or increase tension by placing the band above the knees.

Benefits of Resistance Band Progressions

1. **Continuous Challenge:** Progressions prevent plateaus by challenging muscles with increasing resistance.

2. **Adaptation:** Muscles adapt to increased resistance, leading to improved strength, endurance, and muscle definition.

3. **Customizable Workouts:** Users can easily adjust resistance levels to match their current fitness levels and gradually increase intensity.

Incorporating these advanced techniques and variations into your workout routine provides a dynamic and challenging approach to resistance training. Whether adding resistance bands to traditional exercises or progressing through various resistance levels, these strategies contribute to ongoing muscle development and overall fitness gains. Always prioritize proper form, listen to your body, and progress at a pace that suits your individual fitness level and goals. If needed, seek guidance from a fitness professional to ensure a safe and effective progression plan.

7.3 Loop Band Exercises

Loop bands, also known as mini bands or resistance loops, are small, continuous loops of rubber or fabric designed to be placed around various parts of the body. These bands offer resistance by adding tension to movements and are commonly used for lower body exercises, hip activation, and mobility drills.

Examples of Loop Band Exercises

7.3.1 Glute Bridges with Loop Bands

- *Setup:* Place the loop band just above your knees.

- *Execution:* Perform glute bridges, pushing against the band to engage the glutes and outer thighs.

7.3.2 Lateral Leg Raises with Loop Bands

- *Setup:* Secure the loop band around your ankles.

- *Execution:* Lift one leg sideways against the resistance of the band, targeting the hip abductors.

7.3.3 Monster Walks with Loop Bands

- *Setup:* Position the loop band around your ankles.

- *Execution:* Take lateral steps, maintaining tension on the band, to activate the hip muscles.

Benefits of Loop Band Exercises

1. **Targeted Activation:** Loop bands are particularly effective for activating and strengthening

smaller muscle groups, such as the glutes and hip abductors.

2. **Versatility:** They can be easily incorporated into various exercises and are suitable for both rehabilitation and fitness purposes.

3. **Portability:** Compact and lightweight, loop bands are convenient for home workouts or on-the-go training.

Tube Band Exercises

Definition and Characteristics

Tube bands, also known as resistance tube bands or resistance cords, consist of a flexible tube with handles on each end. These bands offer variable resistance and are suitable for a wide range of exercises targeting both upper and lower body muscles.

Examples of Tube Band Exercises

7.3.4 Bicep Curls with Tube Bands

- *Setup:* Step on the tube band with both feet and hold the handles with your palms facing forward.

- *Execution:* Perform bicep curls, resisting the pull of the band to target the biceps.

7.3.5 Overhead Press with Tube Bands

- *Setup:* Stand on the tube band, holding the handles at shoulder height.

- *Execution:* Press the handles overhead, engaging the shoulders and triceps against the band resistance.

7.3.6 Seated Rows with Tube Bands

- *Setup:* Attach the tube band to a stationary anchor and sit with your legs extended.

- *Execution:* Pull the handles towards your chest, engaging the back muscles.

Benefits of Tube Band Exercises

1. **Variable Resistance:** Tube bands provide variable resistance throughout the range of motion, challenging muscles at different points.

2. **Full-Body Workouts:** Suitable for both upper and lower body exercises, allowing for comprehensive full-body workouts.

3. **Space-Efficient:** Easy to store and transport, making them suitable for home workouts or travel.

7.4 Partner Exercises with Resistance Bands

Partner exercises with resistance bands involve two individuals working together to create resistance and assist in various movements. These exercises add an element of teamwork, motivation, and variability to the workout routine.

Examples of Partner Exercises

7.4.1 Partner Assisted Squats with Resistance Bands

- *Setup:* Both partners stand facing each other with a resistance band looped around their hips.

- *Execution:* Simultaneously perform squats, utilizing the resistance provided by the band.

7.4.2 Banded Partner Rows

- *Setup:* One partner holds the band stationary, while the other performs rows.

- *Execution:* The partner rowing pulls against the resistance provided by the band.

7.4.3 Partner Band Rotations

- *Setup:* Both partners hold opposite ends of a resistance band with arms extended.

- *Execution:* Rotate away from each other, engaging the core and obliques against the band resistance.

Benefits of Partner Exercises with Resistance Bands

1. **Motivation and Accountability:** Partner exercises enhance motivation and accountability, making workouts more enjoyable.

2. **Variability:** Partners can provide different levels of resistance or assistance, allowing for variability in intensity.

3. **Social Interaction:** Partner workouts promote social interaction, creating a sense of camaraderie during exercise.

Incorporating loop band and tube band exercises into your routine provides a versatile and effective means of resistance training. The choice between loop bands and tube bands depends on the specific muscles targeted and the type of exercises desired. Additionally, incorporating partner exercises with resistance bands adds an element of fun and interaction to workouts, fostering a positive and engaging fitness experience. Always ensure proper form and communication during partner exercises to enhance safety and effectiveness.

CHAPTER 8

Creating a Resistance Band Workout Routine

8.1 Designing Beginner, Intermediate, and Advanced Workouts

8.1.1 Beginner Resistance Band Workout

1. **Warm-Up (5 minutes):**

   - Jumping jacks

   - Arm circles

   - Leg swings

2. **Strength Training Circuit (Repeat 2-3 times):**

   - Bodyweight squats: 12 reps

- Resistance band bicep curls: 12 reps

- Band-assisted push-ups: 10 reps

3. **Core Circuit (Repeat 2 times):**

- Plank: 30 seconds

- Russian twists with light band: 12 reps each side

- Seated leg lifts with band: 12 reps

4. **Cool Down (5 minutes):**

- Stretching exercises for major muscle groups

8.1.2 Intermediate Resistance Band Workout

1. **Warm-Up (7 minutes):**

- High knees

- Arm swings

- Dynamic lunges

2. **Strength Training Superset (Repeat 3 times):**

   - Resistance band squats: 15 reps

   - Standing rows with medium band: 12 reps

3. **Upper Body Focus (Repeat 3 times):**

   - Push-ups with resistance band around the back: 12 reps

   - Tricep extensions with band: 15 reps

4. **Core and Stability (Repeat 2 times):**

   - Plank with alternating leg lifts: 45 seconds

   - Pallof press with medium band: 15 reps each side

5. **Cool Down (7 minutes):**

- Stretching and foam rolling for enhanced recovery

8.1.3 Advanced Resistance Band Workout

1. **Warm-Up (10 minutes):**

   - Dynamic movements such as jumping squats and high-intensity intervals

2. **Strength and Power Circuit (Repeat 4 times):**

   - Explosive resistance band deadlifts: 10 reps

   - Medicine ball slams: 15 reps

3. **Full Body Challenge (Repeat 3 times):**

   - Renegade rows with push-ups: 12 reps

   - Tube band jump squats: 20 reps

4. **Advanced Core Circuit (Repeat 3 times):**

- Hanging leg raises with ankle band: 15 reps

- Plank to pike with resistance band around wrists: 10 reps

5. **Cool Down (10 minutes):**

- Yoga-inspired stretches and deep tissue self-myofascial release

8.2 Tips for Progression and Modification

1. **Gradual Resistance Increase:**

- For progression, gradually increase the resistance of your bands as your strength improves.

- Invest in bands with different resistance levels to accommodate various exercises and intensities.

2. **Increase Repetitions or Sets:**

- As you advance, consider adding more repetitions or additional sets to your exercises.

- Be mindful of maintaining proper form and control as you increase the workload.

3. **Vary the Range of Motion:**

- Increase the challenge by incorporating a full range of motion in exercises like squats, lunges, and rows.

- Ensure proper form and control to maximize the benefits and reduce the risk of injury.

4. **Combine Bands for Greater Resistance:**

- Combine multiple bands to create higher resistance

levels for exercises like deadlifts, squats, and rows.

- Securely anchor bands to prevent snapping or slipping during intense workouts.

8.3 Incorporating Resistance Bands into Existing Routines

1. **Warm-Up Activation:**

   - Use light resistance bands for dynamic warm-up exercises, such as leg swings, arm circles, and shoulder rotations, to activate muscles before heavier lifting.

2. **Strength Training:**

   - Replace traditional weights with resistance bands in exercises like squats,

deadlifts, and chest presses
to add variety and challenge
different muscle fibers.

3. **Assisted Pull-Ups and Dips:**

   - Loop a resistance band
     around a pull-up or dip bar
     to assist in these exercises,
     making them more
     accessible for those working
     towards unassisted
     movements.

4. **Core Exercises:**

   - Integrate resistance bands
     into core workouts by
     adding resistance to
     movements like Russian
     twists, bicycle crunches, and
     planks.

5. **Mobility and Stretching:**

   - Use resistance bands to
     enhance stretching and
     improve flexibility. For

example, incorporate band-
assisted stretches for
shoulders, hips, and
hamstrings.

6. **Rehabilitation Exercises:**

- Implement resistance bands
  into rehabilitation routines,
  offering a gentle and
  controlled way to rebuild
  strength after injuries.

By customizing resistance band workouts
to different fitness levels and incorporating
them into existing routines, individuals can
maximize the benefits of these versatile
tools. Consistency, proper form, and
progressive adjustments are key factors in
optimizing the effectiveness of resistance
band workouts. Always listen to your
body, make modifications as needed, and
consult with a fitness professional if you
have specific health concerns or
conditions.

CHAPTER 9

Recovery and Cool Down

9.1 Importance of Cooling Down After Resistance Band Workouts

A cool-down is a crucial component of any workout, including those involving resistance bands. It involves gradually decreasing the intensity of your exercise, helping your body transition from a state of high exertion to a state of rest. Cooling down after a resistance band workout provides several benefits:

1. **Heart Rate Reduction:** Gradually reducing the intensity of exercise helps bring the heart rate back to its resting state, promoting cardiovascular health.

2. **Preventing Dizziness and Lightheadedness:** A cool-down period helps prevent abrupt changes in blood circulation, reducing the risk of dizziness or lightheadedness.

3. **Promoting Flexibility:** Incorporating stretching into the cool-down enhances flexibility, reducing muscle stiffness and promoting a greater range of motion.

4. **Facilitating Waste Product Removal:** Cooling down aids in the removal of metabolic waste products, such as lactic acid, from the muscles, helping prevent soreness and fatigue.

9.2 Stretching Exercises for Post-Workout Recovery

9.2.1 Dynamic Stretching

1. **Leg Swings:**

   - Stand near a support, swing one leg forward and backward in a controlled manner.

   - Repeat 10-15 swings per leg.

2. **Arm Circles:**

   - Extend your arms to the sides and make circular motions in both directions.

   - Perform 1-2 minutes of continuous arm circles.

9.2.2 Static Stretching

1. **Hamstring Stretch:**

   - Sit on the floor with one leg extended and the other bent so the sole of your foot is against the inner thigh.

- Reach for the toes of the extended leg and hold for 15-30 seconds.

2. **Chest Opener:**

   - Stand with feet hip-width apart, clasp your hands behind your back, and lift your arms, opening the chest.

   - Hold for 15-30 seconds.

3. **Quadriceps Stretch:**

   - While standing, bring one heel toward your buttocks, holding the ankle with your hand.

   - Hold for 15-30 seconds per leg.

9.3 Foam Rolling and Self-Myofascial Release Techniques

9.3.1 Foam Rolling

1. **IT Band Roll:**

   - Lie on your side with the foam roller placed under your hip.

   - Roll along the outer thigh, from hip to knee, applying gentle pressure.

2. **Back Roll:**

   - Place the foam roller under your mid-back, supporting your head with your hands.

   - Roll up and down along your upper and mid-back, focusing on areas of tension.

3. **Calf Roll:**

- Sit on the floor with legs extended, placing the foam roller under your calves.

- Roll from the ankles to just below the knees.

9.3.2 Tennis Ball Release

1. **Foot Arch Release:**

   - Place a tennis ball under your foot and roll it back and forth to release tension in the arch.

   - Apply more pressure by pressing your foot onto the ball.

2. **Shoulder Blade Release:**

   - Lie on your back with a tennis ball between your shoulder blade and the floor.

   - Roll side to side to target knots and tight spots.

Benefits of Foam Rolling and Self-Myofascial Release

1. **Improved Flexibility:** Releases tension in the fascia, allowing for improved flexibility and range of motion.

2. **Reduced Muscle Soreness:** Alleviates muscle tightness and soreness by breaking up knots and adhesions.

3. **Enhanced Recovery:** Promotes blood circulation and nutrient flow to muscles, aiding in faster recovery post-exercise.

Incorporating a thorough cool-down, stretching exercises, and foam rolling into your post-resistance band workout routine is essential for optimizing recovery, preventing injury, and promoting overall flexibility and well-being. Prioritize these recovery practices to ensure your body is ready for future workouts and to

experience the full benefits of your
resistance band training.

www.ingramcontent.com/pod-product-compliance
Lightning Source LLC
Chambersburg PA
CBHW070909260726
48661CB00004B/1672